GUIDE TO HEALTHY FOOD

FOR A

HEALTHY BODY

CONTENTS

INTRODUCTION

For some reason, eating healthfully is among the most difficult things a person can accomplish. There are several reasons why eating healthily is difficult, whether it be due to our lack of resources in many areas or the fact that junk food is readily available.

Yes, we can eat almost anything and it will keep us alive. We shall be able to function from one moment to the next and claim to be healthy. But is consuming processed meals and sugary beverages as a sole source of nutrition healthy? We should not assume that just because we are alive, we are healthy. And as we age, our unhealthy behaviors start to catch up with us more and more.

It is crucial to establish healthy eating habits as early as possible in life, if not sooner, in order to avoid problems in the future. You don't want to discover one day that you've been suffering from a vitamin deficit for years and that it's led to consequences that are nearly impossible to treat. We all need to be more accountable for what we put into our bodies since failing to do so can be quite damaging.

Naturally, hindsight is 20/20 when we are older and able to reflect back on our errors. We are aware of the things we could have done—and probably should have done—but didn't because we were either unaware of the negative consequences or were just plain lazy. It's not necessary to act in a health-conscious manner just because you have the knowledge.

In most cases, we don't become more aware of how we treat our bodies and our health in general until we are actually exposed to the misery that can result from poor health decisions. It might be tough to relate to and feel as though the consequences of our actions are extremely far away when we are unable to see their actuality. We might even completely ignore them. Being in this situation can be quite crippling. especially if you are already experiencing the negative impacts of poor eating habits and an unhealthy diet.

Everyone deserves the chance to grow into their best selves, but if we don't even acknowledge the idea that poor eating habits can derail us even in the present, we are eventually saying goodbye to the finest future imaginable.

However, anything can change. You will comprehend the significance of eating healthfully and how food affects our bodies and functions after reading this book.

It can be challenging to stay on track at times if you don't know why your body responds to food the way it does. But there are several ways you might start to comprehend the significance of consuming healthy meals and precisely how to start on a journey toward healthy eating. Let's stop wasting time now. We ought to start eating well right now.

CHAPTER 1: WHY SHOULD I EAT HEALTHY?

There are several reasons why eating healthily is vital. The majority of us are already aware of North America's growing obesity crisis. In general, this is especially true of the United States.

The SAD diet is a term that describes the manner that many Americans eat.

The term "standard American diet," or "SAD," describes a diet that is deficient in nutrition, has a low intake of vegetables, and is rich in fat and sugar.

The SAD diet most likely includes processed foods. These are quick, simple, and readily available foods that have detrimental long-term impacts on health.

Avoiding such processed meals and focusing instead on whole grains, fruits, vegetables, and meat that has not been treated with hormones or other chemicals that may ultimately find their way into your body and create problems is generally regarded as a good option if you want to prevent being obese. Unfortunately, there are many opportunities in North America for us to put off cooking meals.

We have so many items at our disposal, and purchasing poor quality food costs far less than purchasing high quality food. It may seem unusual that buying organic costs more than buying foods that may eventually lead to long-term health issues, but supply and demand dictate that this is the case.

Additionally, due to their ease, processed foods are mass-produced and extremely profitable. Because of this, the obesity pandemic in North America is not entirely unexpected. On the list of businesses aiming to profit from people's lack of interest in cooking, nutrition is not at the top.

However, there are numerous benefits to eating well and compelling arguments against following the typical American diet and processed foods. For instance, you should absolutely check into the rest of this book to find strategies to modify your nutrition and start a healthy lifestyle if you do not want to be obese.

By consuming unhealthy foods and adhering to the typical American diet, which is high in fat and sugar, you might increase your risk of contracting diseases. Diabetes is a condition that can arise by eating poorly and is frequently treated with a good diet.

In the end, type II diabetes is something that can be maintained and treated with healthy eating habits and is something that is started by unhealthy eating habits. Make an effort to make wise eating decisions if you wish to stay away from these kinds of challenges and complication.

Poor eating can also lead to other ailments. Both chronic illnesses like high blood pressure and others are widespread.

Because they didn't make proper food decisions earlier in life, osteoporosis is something that can afflict many people later in life. You can experience cardiac issues, high blood pressure, or poor bone health. All of which put a lot of stress on your body and can be extremely dangerous in the long run.

You should start making decisions now that will enable you to remain in their life for as long as possible if you want to demonstrate to your family that you care about them. Your poor health doesn't just affect you. It is something that also has an impact on those close to you. In a way, it is rather selfish if people are watching you suffer as a result of your terrible decisions. They are also in pain. Do your best right now to choose what will ultimately be best for your family as well as yourself. This book will demonstrate how.

CHAPTER 2: UNDERSTANDING HOW YOU RELATED TO FOOD

Everybody starts to acquire certain habits over time. We form habits in every area of our lives. We form a variety of habits, including ones related to eating, sleeping, and working. However, until they start to have a detrimental impact on us, they are typically fairly unaware of our habits. Even still, it can be very challenging to modify our habits once we start to realize how negatively our habits are affecting us. Since I have that, that is how it is.

We often act almost subconsciously when we have a habit. It takes a lot of willpower to break free from the cycle because these habits are ingrained in us.

It becomes much simpler to change your thinking once you realize that your connection with food has everything to do with the habits you have formed and can continue to form.

When you are aware of the significance of your future and the impact and necessity of making wise decisions on these matters, you may be more motivated to engage in healthy eating and less likely to do actions that may harm you in the long run.

To be honest, it seems that many of us see a gloomy future. Because it is irrelevant whether we make wise decisions or not if we do not think we have anything positive to look forward to, we do not perceive sufficient reasons to modify our patterns.

We do not see how we can genuinely shape the future in a way that is beneficial to us. We probably don't believe we have any control over our life because of this.

Don't be concerned if you can identify with this emotion. The human experience is incredibly common. Since we are frequently instructed what to do by others, we are typically discouraged from asserting our authority and using our power from a young age. In some cases, we even stop believing that we have any control over our life.

That makes sense when you're a kid. It's not always obvious to kids what's best for them. But it could also promote a highly powerless mindset, which makes it difficult for us to see how much our behavior's results can actually influence who we are and how we come across to others.

To properly understand yourself and your eating patterns, you must therefore take the necessary actions. What year did your habit start? How did you get into that routine? Why? What advantages do you get from this practice? What unfavorable consequences does this habit cause you?

Ask yourself as many of these inquiries as you can so that you may start to comprehend how your present and future are being shaped by the food you consume.

Are you constructing a future that is energetic and healthy, or are you constructing one that is hopeless and might contain many unfavorable health effects?

Assess your level of self-discipline next. Can you use self-control when making decisions? Or do you find it difficult in this area? Everybody can struggle with discipline, therefore if you are one of those people, you should consider how you can motivate yourself to be more self-disciplined both in your daily life and in your thoughts.

You won't be ready to start your journey toward healthy eating until then. Because poor health decisions are available everywhere, whether we like it or not. Both simple and addictive, they are.

It won't matter whether you occasionally eat nutritious food or not if we allow ourselves to be influenced by these bad decisions and don't change our routines. The harmful consequences will continue to grip your body and wait for an opportunity to manifest themselves when you least expect it.

Unhealthy eating is, in a sense, a pattern of self-destruction that many of us engage in. Self-destructive eating habits are risky, whether they result from low self-esteem or are only a result of dissatisfaction with the

11

present and lack of hope for the future. Prior to making healthy eating a habit, you must look inward and genuinely respect your life and your future.

You can accomplish this in a variety of ways, and if necessary, you might even want to seek the assistance of a mental health expert. They occasionally assist us in identifying biases and unfavorable trends in our life that we are unaware of. Once you've acknowledged and recognized them, it may be much simpler to move past them and take the necessary actions to make wise decisions.

There are many things you can do to alter your thinking, regardless of whether you seek the assistance of a trained expert or not.

You will be willing to make the required efforts to achieve your goals as long as you believe that you are deserving of a healthy body and a promising future.

But it will be more tougher if you don't feel good about yourself. In general, you will be helped on your trip if you can understand yourself, your habits, your mental barriers, and your discipline. Healthy eating is a fantastic start in the path of being the best version of ourselves for each and every one of us to take every day. Furthermore, we can do it right now!

CHAPTER 3: DIET TRENDS AND THEIR RISKS

Today's society is rife with diet trends, and almost all of them are associated with risks. Sadly, most people who are eager to make money frequently fail to consider the long-term health effects of their products. They are primarily focused on making money and doing things that will enable them to take advantage of the desperate need that many people have to lose weight quickly and easily.

If diet trends are something that pique your attention, there is something that you will have to accept. Unfortunately, there is no good technique to lose weight quickly and effortlessly without effort, a nutritious diet, or exercise. If you are overweight or in need of more mobility due to insufficient fitness, losing weight is a desirable objective.

We can all agree that sometimes we need to start living healthier lives. Instead of putting our trust in businesses that wish to take advantage of us in order to profit, we can achieve this by eating well and moving our bodies.

Some of the current eating trends are extremely harmful and have severe short- and long-term health effects. Many of them rely on techniques that deprive Robert's body and ourselves of vital nutrients. even dehydrating us at times.

These diet fads are abhorrent in every way. They are preying on those who desire health but lack the knowledge to get it. They prey on individuals, frequently women in particular, who are breaking under the weight of unattainable beauty standards and who are convinced that in order to be considered valuable, they need to appear a specific way.

That is wholly false. You have worth whether you are 100 or 700 pounds. However, eating healthily is one of the few effective methods you'll be able to jump-start your metabolism and provide your body the nutrition it needs to operate at its peak potential.

If you deprive your body of the vitamins and minerals it needs to survive and rely on a diet fad to teach you how to slim down and feel good when all they actually want is your cash, you'll finish up more behind than you were when you started. The unpleasant reality is that many diet fads send the body into famine mode.

Your metabolism could be damaged by this, which would make you gain weight more quickly in the future. Don't let the advertising that claim to make weight loss quick and simple take advantage of you. All of that will be expensive. Additionally, there are health fads out there, like the hCG diet, that can seriously mess with your body and hormones.

Diet trends are hilarious in that they frequently lead to unhealthy and challenging methods of weight maintenance, which will make it more difficult for you to lose weight in the future. Do not believe a drug you see advertised on television if you want to lose weight. Replace unhealthy processed and sugary foods with whole-grain alternatives and organic fruits and vegetables to avoid introducing chemicals into your body that will make it more difficult for you to lose weight and ultimately disrupt your body chemistry.

It may be alluring to be able to lose weight rapidly without having to give up the unhealthy eating habits you have accumulated over the years, but this is unhealthy. If you are not careful about how you try to reduce weight, you are harming yourself and setting up your body for future health issues. Aim to make decisions that you would like other people to make for themselves by doing everything in your ability to do so.

Before you succumb to the TV snake oil salesman, do some homework. Look into these matters because you deserve a bright future and you are worth doing things the correct way, not one that is complicated by the negative effects of a sales pitch that only cares about your wallet and not your health.

CHAPTER 4: THE FOOD PYRAMYD

The food pyramid has most likely been seen by all of us. The food pyramid was frequently used as a reference point for us as children to give us an idea of how much and what kind of food we should eat on a daily basis in order to maintain a healthy lifestyle.

Of course, there is always proof that the food pyramid is flexible, but overall, if you can follow the food pyramid, you'll have a rough understanding of what constitutes a balanced, healthy diet.

Even if this is occasionally debatable, it's nevertheless beneficial to eat some staples. Maybe one that you come up with yourself. Many people would assert that eating as many grains as the food pyramid may have recommended is no longer thought to be the healthiest course of action.

In fact, many people are promoting a no-grain lifestyle as the healthiest option in light of recent celiac disease outbreaks.

Try to evaluate your own unique experiences with food before depending on the food pyramid as your fundamental guideline for what is healthy to eat, and go from there. With a lot of grains, some people are healthier, while others are not. To the best of your ability, use your judgment in this situation so that you can move in the appropriate way for your health.

The traditional food pyramid suggests the following:

You should have between three and five portions of vegetables and fruits each day, but you can consume up to 11 servings of rice, cereal, pasta, and bread.

When it comes to meet and beans, as well as other foods like nuts and fish or poultry, it is advised that you have two or three servings every day. Unsurprisingly, things like sugar and fat and oil are the very tip of the.

As far as their eggs, you can have two or three servings every day, provided you are not allergic to or lactose intolerant. Because you shouldn't have too much of any of these. Instead, utilize them sparingly to ensure that you are leading the healthiest lifestyle possible.

Once more, this is merely a reference to the conventional food pyramid.

You may need to alter this chart to suit your particular needs and dietary requirements. This is the norm for the food pyramid, however, that can be used to your fullest advantage in order to develop a healthier lifestyle if you do not have any particular needs.

CHAPTER 5: USING FOOD AS MEDICATION

In the same way that eating poorly can make you unwell, eating well can frequently make you feel better and help you recover from illness.

Additionally, it can be used as a defense against disease.

In truth, Aryuveda, a comprehensive healing system, has been practiced in India for thousands of years.

This age-old method of treatment is used to treat any condition by just altering your diet. The food that has kept Indians alive for so many years is essentially their medication. And it might still be relevant today.

As a matter of fact, many cures are nothing more than wholesome meals with anti-inflammatory characteristics and the capacity to nourish your body from the inside out. Healthy food choices have been shown to have an impact on anything from cancer to infections.

And that has never been more clear than with this traditional healing technique.

However, a lot of it has been tried and true for thousands of years and will continue to have an impact on the body. Of course, a lot of current technology will disapprove of these methods because they have not been properly researched.

Food can ultimately determine whether or not you are susceptible to illness, whether or not you believe in the ancient healing art. Your body will be stronger and more capable of fighting off disease and infection if you eat well than it would be if you were undernourished and following the typical American diet.

Fighting off the unpleasant consequences of disease can be nearly impossible if your body lacks the necessary vitamins and minerals.

It may occasionally even result in disease. Certain types of poor unprocessed foods might cause illnesses and increase your risk of developing certain cancers if you eat them often.

Despite the fact that scientists are continually learning more about cancer and do not yet have a complete understanding of how to cure it, there are several examples of people who were able to live long, healthy lives by just making the necessary lifestyle changes.

A healthy diet can aid in reducing the symptoms of numerous ailments that are difficult and/or incurable, such as multiple sclerosis.

They will continue to do this as long as you make sure that everything you put into your body is nourishing and giving your organs and cells all of the fuel and resources they require to keep your body strong. And they'll try their hardest to succeed.

However, if you are deliberately harming your body, it won't be able to fight back as well as it could if it were well nourished. Because of this, it is crucial that you pay attention to how you are feeding your body. You may be setting yourself up for failure in ways that you may later come to regret if you do not actively and consciously choose the food that you consume.

CHAPTER 6: EATING VEGETABLES HAS HEALTH BENEFITS

One of the most underrated foods in the world is vegetables, particularly when it comes to the typical American diet. Most people are unaware of how crucial it is to give the body the vitamins and minerals that only veggies and vegetables alone can offer. When it comes to enhancing their appearance, people occasionally show an interest in vegetables, but they lose that desire when it comes to enhancing their health.

But since you are here and reading this book, it is safe to assume that you are able and willing to consider the benefits of eating veggies. The best justifications for including veggies in your diet on a regular basis are listed below.

First and foremost, fiber helps the body get rid of extra waste. Without a way to be combined and expelled, waste builds up inside the body and can lead to weight gain and other problems.

There are numerous additional benefits of fiber. It can assist you in preventing an increase in your blood cholesterol and even help you avoid heart disease or at least reduce your risk of developing it.

Folic acid is a molecule that is also found in vegetables, and when you give it to your body, it can help your body produce red blood cells.

21

This can be particularly good for women in particular, who often need this chemical during pregnancy and menstruation, and it can be very significant in assisting you in preventing anemia from arising.

Additionally, vegetables naturally include a lot of vitamins, including vitamins A and C, which aid in infection prevention and overall wellness. Another strategy to treat and prevent anemia from arising is by increasing your ability to absorb iron and speed up the healing process. Potassium is a very important component of vitamins because it keeps the body from developing excessive blood pressure.

There is evidence that eating more vegetables lowers the risk of stroke and other heart-related problems. They can stop the formation of kidney stones and stop bone tissue from deteriorating. Consuming plenty of vegetables will help you control type II diabetes and obesity.

In addition, it may provide you the strength you need to battle cancer and avoid it. Eating veggies has several benefits, but one of the best is probably that they are very low in fat and definitely low in calories.

This indicates that you don't need to worry too much about gaining weight if you eat a lot of vegetables.

Vegetables are a terrific snack since they can help you control your appetite and maintain your commitment to living a healthy lifestyle.

Vegetables are fantastic in so many ways. It is unexpected that they are so scarce in the typical American diet.

Walking around your grocery store's exterior first is one of the finest things you can do to assist yourself avoid processed foods that are heavy in fat, sugar, and salt.

Instead of skipping to the end and cheating by buying pastas and other processed meals that are poor in actually nutritious vegetable content, make purposeful decisions to provide your body with healthy fresh vegetable selections by moving along the fresh produce department.

Making choices that will fuel your body is the first step in healthy eating, and veggies are among the most nourishing foods.

Inadequate eating habits early in life or even self-imposed ones later on can cause us to lose our taste for healthy foods, but it is simple to get back on track. Give vegetables a place in your life. The advantages may require a little more time to prepare, but they are worthwhile.

CHAPTER 7: EATING FRUITS HAS HEALTH BENEFITS

People who consume the typical American diet do not consume enough fruit, which is a sad but well-known fact. They typically eat fruit that is either in cans or that has been heavily sweetened.

The body cannot receive any health advantages from consuming fruit in its natural state because of the added sugar and fruit.

Consuming excessive amounts of fruit might have certain drawbacks, particularly if you have diabetes. Fruit is rich in natural sugars, and juicing it yields a large amount of sugar without much fiber, which might give the body an excess.

Fruit is one of the healthiest foods because it contains fiber, which lowers heart disease risk and prevents constipation. Furthermore, meals high in fiber, such as fruits and vegetables, are excellent for controlling weight because they make you feel full on fewer calories. Fruit is also a good source of several vitamins and minerals, particularly vitamin C, which is particularly abundant in citrus fruits.

When it comes to promoting the body's ability to heal, vitamin C is a force to be reckoned with, and fruits high in the vitamin will do the trick if you want to maintain the health of your teeth and gums.

Fruit can also aid in the prevention of kidney stones and strokes, two additional goals for the body. Fruits are incredibly beneficial for strengthening the body and preventing and treating diseases including skin concerns and heart issues. Fruit can be one of the healthiest methods to give you a boost of energy and satisfy any sugar cravings you may experience as a result of trying to eliminate bad items from your diet.

You can have a nutritious snack that fulfills your sweet taste if you are willing to take use of the incredible power of fruit, as long as you aren't going overboard with your fruits, such as putting a lot of them in the blender and ultimately consuming an absurd quantity of sugar.

Fruits and vegetables both naturally have a propensity to make your skin glow and appear considerably more hydrated and nourished, which is good news if you're interested in the health benefits that food can provide. Fruits and vegetables are rich in antioxidants, vitamins, and minerals that give your body the water it needs to maintain a youthful appearance and good skin.

Along with keeping your skin looking young, it can help your hair grow out softer and healthier. Fruit can even assist you in halting acne in its tracks by moisturizing your face and keeping your body clear of waste materials that exit through your pores. You will rapidly start to notice the advantages of that aspect of fruit because of its high water content, which is beneficial for helping the body keep hydrated.

Additionally, fruit is particularly beneficial for digestion.

Due to its high fiber content, it aids in the binding of waste and aids the body in getting rid of items that could otherwise be problematic.

As a result, eating fruit and vegetables can help you lose weight.

The body gets rid of waste before it has a chance to break down and be stored as fat.

You can also prevent and fight disease, including cancer, by eating fruit. Some fruits, like apples, can prevent asthma attacks. The cholesterol levels of others can be dramatically reduced.

Additionally, grapes—particularly red-skinned grapes—have been reported to be employed in the fight against cancer. Additionally, they are beneficial in the treatment of kidney and eye conditions. Berries are particularly useful if you have an infection. Antioxidants are abundant in them.

To avoid complications with weight loss and health problems, only eat fruits and vegetables that have not been exposed to commercial pesticides. These foods can absorb pesticides and make it more difficult to lose weight.

To give your body a sweet snack that will be incredibly nutritious, you can even consume dry fruits in place of harmful and sugary snacks. Just be mindful of the sugar content in dried fruits because, occasionally, when they are commercially offered, added sugars transform what could be a nutritious treat into something that may ultimately contribute to you gaining weight.

However, fruit might assist you in losing weight if you consume it regularly and in a healthy manner. The fibers and water in fruit will make your body feel full and replenish your cells and organs, so long as you are not overeating foods with a lot of sugar. You will experience a significant change in your energy levels overall, and the fiber and water content will assist you in removing problems that are causing obesity.

This energy can be used to workout and strive even harder for a healthy lifestyle. As you continue to make the move toward greater health and wellbeing, this can be particularly beneficial if you're substituting sugary junk food with healthy fruit substitutes.

CHAPTER 8: DISCUSSES THE HEALTHIEST MEAT TO CONSUME

Although it may come as a surprise to learn that there are some meats that are healthier than others, meat is typically thought of as one of the main staple items in an email. Of course, we are aware of the distinction between red and white meats. White meats are generally seen to be leaner and healthier overall, whereas red meat is more frequently associated with health difficulties and cardiovascular disorders.

Some folks might be surprised to learn that meats also have other health risks. issues including what the animals are given while they are still alive and possible injections of antibiotics and hormones to hasten their growth or increase their milk production, at least in the case of cows.

These hormones can harm our bodies by eventually making their way into the meat we eat. If we are careless with the decisions we make while selecting our foods, they may eventually lead to poor health in the future, including but not limited to tumors and hormone changes that can be very debilitating.

However, if you are sure that the sources of your meat are safe and do not overfeed animals with steroids and antibiotics, you are already one step ahead of the game. If so, try doing some research on local establishments where you can get meat that hasn't been tainted by any hazardous industrial standards.

Nevertheless, even when taking into account the selection of healthy meats, some meats are healthier than others. In particular if you want to reduce weight, fish is one of the healthiest meats you can eat. Fish is full of nutrients and lean. Regarding the origin of your fish, you must take care.

Some fish are grown in unsanitary conditions, while other fish may originate from regions that could be mercury-contaminated. For this reason, eating fish or shellfish while pregnant is not advised.

However, fish can be really nutritious for your body if you can find a good source of it. Fish has a lot of omega-3 fatty acids, which are good for your memory and brain health. Overall, omega three fatty acids are widely sought-after and necessary for optimal body function, particularly when it comes to mental processes.

A fantastic alternative is chicken that has been grown in a healthy setting. Chicken has a lot of protein. In actuality, it has the highest protein content of any type of meat. They are typically raised under favorable circumstances, or at the very least fed diets that won't harm humans' bodies in the same way as eating a lot of beef may.

However, if you are consuming grass-fed beef from a reliable source, it might also be a fantastic choice. There are typically fewer chances that the chicken you eat was reared with harmful carcinogens if it was organic.

When hens are raised conventionally, they are frequently offered substances that speed up their growth, which can have detrimental effects on both the health of the chickens and the people who eat them. Additionally, a lot of painkillers, antidepressants, and occasionally even arsenic and caffeine are given to them.

It is dangerous to consume a lot of meat from conventionally raised animals, but if you can locate a reliable supplier, you should do it.

Because it has a lot of selenium, turkey is another excellent meat. The body will benefit greatly from this, especially as it can aid in the removal of toxins and free radicals.

However, you should still make an effort to ensure that the meat you eat comes from reliable sources because it is customary for conventionally grown chicken and turkey to be treated similarly and fed dangerous chemicals that unnaturally accelerate their rate of growth and ultimately contaminate human bodies with those chemicals.

Overall, eating meat may be highly healthy for the body, as long as you avoid consuming any that was raised using risky or unnatural techniques. The poisons that these animals are frequently exposed to are extremely harmful to both the animals and the people that consume them.

Avoiding substances that might remain in your body and stop weight loss from happening is preferable if you want to eat healthily and lose weight.

Even if you don't want to lose weight, eating healthily entails staying away from anything that could be harmful to the body, such as hormones and chemicals that can upset our delicate systems. If you want to indulge in chicken, beef, or even lamb, there are fortunately several of choices for healthy meats.

You can satisfy any cravings you may have with ethically produced, wholesome food.

CHAPTER 9: THE RISKS OF PROCESSED FOODS

Anyone who has ever consumed processed food is aware of their hazard. The fact that they are still permitted to be on the shelves, despite the damage they cause to our bodies and minds, is surprising. For some people, choosing to eat poorly is more than just a personal preference.

People in poverty are occasionally compelled to turn to processed meals since they offer an affordable and simple solution to feed large families on a tight budget due to the way the economy operates.

The difficult part of that is that these foods ultimately result in medical issues down the road that cost even more money than it would to feed a large family with healthy, sustainable options. In the end, it appears that those with less resources are suffering in either case.

Processed meals are simply unhealthy, even if you don't need to feed a family on a tight budget. They include a lot of fat and sugar, which contributes to their addictive nature.

They are frequently packed meals with a lot of sugar and pasta in them. In general, too much sugar is harmful, but for those who are predisposed to type II diabetes in particular. If you consume sugar frequently and in large amounts, your body will eventually become overloaded, and you will likely not only grow obese but also have other health problems.

Due to the fact that sugar increases insulin resistance, which makes it harder, if not impossible, to control your blood sugar levels, sugar can assist hasten the development of diabetes.

There will undoubtedly be a detrimental effect if you consume these meals frequently, such as at every meal or at the very least every day.

Regularly consuming that much fat and sugar can cause heart disease, cancer, diabetes, and other illnesses besides the well-known ones like obesity and diabetes. Processed foods should be avoided at all costs because this is extremely harmful.

Eating processed foods has the additional drawback of being exceedingly artificial and addictive. The majority of the elements in those foods don't nourish the body in any way. Instead, they are making us feel full while depriving our bodies of the necessary nutrients for normal operation.

We ultimately enable ourselves to become more simple-minded when we consume bland, unnourishing foods. We are not functioning to the best of our abilities in terms of thinking, moving, and overall performance. All of these items are very harmful and may result in sluggish coordination and even melancholy.

On some level, we can all agree that processed meals are less healthier than the kinds of things we should be eating frequently. Even if our minds are unaware, our bodies are aware of it. As a result, we suffer. It's causing us stress.

Whether we are addicted to them or not, our bodies are aware when we overindulge in harmful meals. We frequently punish ourselves, whether it's unconsciously done or not. We are aware that we are misbehaving. Even if we are now processing it, we feel angry and unsatisfied about it.

Additionally, processed meals contain a lot of artificial colorings, which have been shown to be very carcinogenic. We essentially ingest dye when we eat foods that have fixed coloring in them. Do you think you could eat hair dye? Really not. However, your food contains these kinds of substances. They don't leave your body; they stay inside. Inside, they color your inside organs.

They are extremely harmful and can cause cancer.

Preservatives abound in them as well. The shelf life of processed food is very long. more time than is healthy or typical. The usual milk bottle would not last for months on end.

It would curdle and deteriorate. the same as with cheeses and other goods that are available on store shelves and have a long shelf life.

Companies must determine shelf life since they may generate more revenue if their food can be kept on the shelf for an extended period of time. To ensure that they are earning the most money possible, they will do whatever it takes, regardless of whether it is healthier or less harmful to the human body.

Preservatives frequently contain toxic, synthetic substances and excessive salt. Both of which are detrimental to the body in some way. Because they contain an excessive amount of salt, processed meals can induce hypertension and heart problems. Among North America, obesity and heart attacks are among the leading causes of death, and high blood pressure is a regular occurrence in persons who live solely off of processed foods.

The typical American diet is largely responsible for this. The terrible thing is that these processed meals are incredibly addictive even if you are aware of their unhealthiness due to their high chemical, sugar, and fat content.

It can be almost as harmful as developing a drug addiction because the body starts to want them. Your health and development may suffer long-term effects if you become addicted to a diet that is neither nourishing nor healthy.

Because humans digest processed foods far more quickly than foods high in beneficial dietary fiber, they also contribute to obesity. We may not even be expending as much energy as we would when digesting nutritious foods if we are digesting these foods quickly and they are not filling us up because we are not getting the fiber that gives us the feeling of being full.

This implies that we eat more and digest less, which causes a quick and rapid increase in weight. When you consume a diet high in processed foods, your body contains significantly more calories. When you eat wholesome, high-dietary fiber foods, you burn a lot more calories than you otherwise would.

Sadly, this means that whether they intend to or not, people who live and thrive on a diet of processed foods will eventually gain weight. Additionally, because they don't nourish you, they won't provide you as much energy.

As a result, you consume a lot more of these harmful, sugar-rich meals without feeling satisfied or full, which is likely to leave you feeling drained, lethargic, and way too full.

Our bodies are unable to adequately process processed meals. They quickly convert to fat. Furthermore, they contain a lot of fat.

They frequently contain sugars and fats that are disguised. High fructose corn syrup, a major contributor to weight gain, is one of the main ingredients in many of these processed foods, along with vegetable oil.

Given that the majority of processed foods on the market contain high fructose corn syrup, it is understandable why North America is currently experiencing the largest obesity pandemic in recorded history.

Due to their inability to degrade, hydrogenated oils are very unhealthy.

They stay in your body and mix with your fat cells.

These oils make burning fat much more challenging. These fat deposits are more difficult to lose, and they can quickly cause obesity. Most of the nutritional value required by humans for optimal function is not included in the ingredients of processed foods. Before we can completely thrive, we require the fibers, vitamins, and minerals that are included in actual food.

If eating processed foods can't be completely avoided, at least consume them in moderation. They are perilous.

They can generally make us feel down, angry, and sad.

When we switch from a healthy diet to one that consists mostly of processed foods that are too sweet, too fatty, and too unhealthy, our dispositions may shift from favorable to unfavorable.

Our bodies yearn for nourishment. Providing your body with that nutrition is the simplest and most advantageous thing you can do for yourself. It can be challenging to adjust to new routines, such surviving solely on processed foods, and it can be extremely unpleasant at times.

Spending more time in the kitchen preparing and thinking about your meals and health is required. But in the end, consuming manufactured meals can cause your death and sever your connection to yourself. Instead of giving your body an opportunity to get rid of the garbage you are putting into it, you are really absorbing poisons and avoiding nutrients that can act as antioxidants.

Junk food and processed food are the same thing. The same applies to them. They resemble junk food yet seem healthier. In reality, they are nibbles. The first and most effective step you can take to get healthy and genuinely feel healthy is to avoid processed meals at all costs. Don't be duped by the packaging that suggests these items are healthful.

They lack everything that nourishes your body and are high in salt, sugar, and saturated fat. Make every effort to break your reliance on processed meals. If you make the effort, eating well is simple and doable.

Just keep in mind to avoid the aisles that are full of harmful and seductive packaging that conceals the risks of the processed food inside by strolling around the grocery store to pick up the fresh produce and meat instead.

CHAPTER 10: USING MEAL PLANNING TO TIE EVERYTHING TOGHETER

One of the key elements in establishing a healthy lifestyle is meal planning. It can be very simple to give in to the temptations of unhealthily addictive meals when we are unable to envision the future of our diet. especially if it has become our habit to eat them instead of nourishing foods.

It takes a lot of work to arrange meals. For someone who struggles with organizing, it can be a little scary. Do not worry if you find it difficult to plan your meals. Whether you lack creativity in the kitchen or not, there are numerous simple and enjoyable ways for you to start preparing your meals.

There are numerous meal planning packages available for purchase. Many of them provide the possibility to order boxes filled with fresh ingredients for cooking that also come with usable recipes. This is frequently the case if you are not accustomed to cooking.

In particular when it seems challenging to carve out the time necessary to prepare substantial, nutritional meals due to bad eating habits and a hectic work schedule. Research is done as the initial stage in meal planning. If you want to become healthier, you need to consider your options.

The best way to begin is by researching recipes. It can be entertaining and educational to compile a binder of nutritious meals that you want to try. You might learn stuff you didn't know before, or it might open your eyes to a variety of cuisine options you might have previously laughed off as being out of your league in terms of difficulty to make.

Recipes have a way of opening our minds. Particularly when you are eager to learn new things. It can be challenging to develop the habit of cooking, but once you do, you'll be astonished at how much freedom you'll discover in creating a dinner for yourself that is both nutritious and delectable!

Get a collection of recipes you wish to try by looking through cookbooks and publications. If you are a beginner in the kitchen, you could also want to start with the dishes that appear to be the most straightforward. Begin with the foods that appear to be the most appetizing and nourishing.

The next step is to maintain a straightforward, user-friendly organization for your recipes. Meal planning will be made more challenging if you start to feel disorganized and overwhelmed.

Making sure that everything is as simple as possible while starting a new habit is important. You should always aim to introduce tiny, simple modifications until they have established a new habit because too much change at once might be stressful on your system.

So that you can immediately start making your supper when you want to, make sure they are nearby and accessible. If you're using a binder, you might want to think about laminating the pages or using plastic sleeves so that, if you're using it in the kitchen, they won't get contaminated by water or other food.

It would be beneficial to arrange your recipes in the sequence of breakfast dishes, lunch dishes, supper dishes, and snacks.

Once you start cooking, this will make it easier for you to refer to the appropriate recipes. If you'd like, you could even arrange your binder according to the days of the week, including printed copies of your daily meal plans.

You could arrange your recipes in a variety of ways. Follow your intuition and do what feels right. Do not force yourself to stick to a structure that is not effective for you. Make sure you are doing what is best for you in your own life, instead.

To keep your imagination flowing and your kitchen exciting, make sure you are making the time to periodically look for new recipes that stand out to you. There are many different kinds of dishes you may try, and the more you do, the more exciting eating healthily can be!

The next thing you should do is look at Microsoft Office programs like Excel that can assist you in organizing your food planning. There are numerous templates available on Excel that you may use to organize your meals by day, time, and week. This is potentially a very useful tool!

There are apps available for your phone, tablet, or other device that you may download if you'd prefer not to use Excel to help you make better use of your time and resources.

Even better, you can go the traditional method and get a notebook made just for making meal plans. Making your meals accessible and organized requires you to take one crucial step.

When starting a journey toward healthy eating, a meal plan is really helpful. You will inevitably fall up at some point as developing excellent habits requires time and patience.

You're not need to remain rooted to the ground, though!

The truth is that it just means you have to get back up and keep trying, as giving up is far simpler than sticking to your intentions.

Remaining consistent with the theme can be a big help when it comes to meal planning. People frequently have special themes, such as Taco Tuesday or another day designated for a particular kind of dish. Feel free to follow suit with that kind of meal planning if you believe it will keep you on track. Because it works and keeps things straightforward and organized, it is done for a reason.

If you want to keep things simple, that can be a fantastic approach to go about it. It can be really unpleasant to find yourself forced to do a lot of planning and preparation every single week or month. You may alternate between a biweekly meal plan with a theme, such as taco Tuesday one night and perhaps rice and vegetables Tuesday the following. Planning your meals can be done in any way. Follow through must be observed, and this is what you must do.

Everything else becomes unnecessary and difficult without follow-through. Accountability is something that may really assist you in making meal planning a success. Ask someone you like and care about if they would be willing to help you stick to your schedule if you let them know that you are trying to plan daily meals.

By enquiring about your progress and whether you are staying on course, they can be of assistance to you. They could also decide to support you and cheer you on in your achievements.

They can be quite beneficial for both of you, regardless of how they decide to assist you. Knowing that you have supporters in your corner who genuinely want you to succeed can be wonderful if they are a positive and encouraging individual. Just be careful to get rid of toxic people who make you feel inferior by drawing attention to themselves or by giving you the impression that it will be challenging for you to achieve your objectives.

Constructive criticism can be quite helpful, but if you aren't looking for it, it can also be harmful.

Make sure you know the difference between a toxic individual who poses as supportive and a supportive person who genuinely wants you to succeed.

Taking personal responsibility is another approach to accept accountability. Journaling and self-affirmations can help you become more accountable to yourself. Talking to yourself about your objectives, whether internally or aloud, can be a helpful method to keep motivated and assess whether you are taking the actions you want to take.

If you discover that you are not, rather than criticizing yourself, take into account your barriers and continue on as you start to identify them. Only if you never try will you ever be a failure.

Everything will eventually fall into place if you try since you are putting out the effort and making positive changes in your life.

There are several benefits to keeping a journal. You can use their assistance to remember what, when, and how much you've eaten. This will give you a decent notion of what you may expect from yourself in terms of reality. You need to address and make a note of the things you are not happy with. But rather than getting frustrated with yourself for not being a trickle right away, keep in mind that it is a process and you need to move carefully.

Start slowly by easing into one or two meals a week instead of imposing a complete shift in routine and scheduling every meal for the next month when you have never done it before. As you become more familiar with the procedure, gradually add in the remaining meals.

Make sure it won't startle you in any way. The most enduring change is gradual. Additionally, writing about your experiences in a notebook may help you explore your deepest feelings regarding the procedure and any obstacles you might not have even been aware of.

As your conduct starts to take on patterns, you may be able to anticipate when and why you might be inclined to stray from your course. It will be simpler to steer clear of them in the future if you can recognize these trigger points.

Organizing your meals may be a lot of fun and thrilling. Even if you don't love that level of organization, it can be incredibly gratifying to consider exactly what you will be putting in your body and to take the necessary measures to make that happen. With meal planning and a good helping of self-esteem, you will be well on your way to a lifestyle of healthy eating. Everyone deserves the chance to become the healthiest and most nutritious version of themselves.

CONCLUSION

It can be really challenging to start eating healthily, especially if you were not able to form healthy eating habits as a young child. It is feasible to develop a stronger sense of health awareness and proactivity, though.

Fortunately, we can start improving ourselves and moving forward in life each and every day that we wake up breathing.

Being the best version of ourselves can first seem scary, but as you begin to understand that every decision you make affects your life—whether positively or negatively—it gets much simpler to see where our actions are going before they come back to bite us. Poor dietary decisions will undoubtedly haunt us in the future.

If we are careless about what we put into our bodies while we are younger, we risk starting to experience health issues later in life. The only way to cultivate a healthy and happy body and mind is via good food and exercise.

When we are confined to our houses all day, consuming only processed meals high in sugar and fat, and sitting around watching TV without exercising, we start to get restless and stir crazy. People's lives are being lost as a result of the risky American diet. Don't allow yourself turn into one of them.

Make the decisions you need to in order to actually improve yourself and develop into the best version of yourself instead.

Make decisions that will honor your family and ensure that they can count on you for many years to come.

This is truly very selfish when we don't look after ourselves. Whether we are aware of it or not, there are individuals in our immediate vicinity who genuinely care about the people we are and the value we add to their lives. Everyone should have the opportunity to shape their own future and make decisions that will help them for many years to come.

One approach to start bettering yourself and preparing your body and mind for the future is through healthy nutrition.

Healthy eating is something that you should start doing as soon as possible if you want to be independent and active for as long as you can without spending yourself thousands upon thousands of dollars in medical bills and other expenses.

If not, it will inevitably become a financial and physical burden on your life. You are now better equipped to start living a healthy lifestyle after reading this book and using the advice it contains.

Your quality of life will be significantly improved both now and in the future if you plan your meals and learn more about why it is crucial to make healthy food choices. The benefits of healthy eating will start to become apparent as soon as you maintain your commitment! You only need to try. You are capable of completing this.